EXERCISE AND PHYSICAL ACTIVITY FOR SENIORS WITH STAGE 3 KIDNEY DISEASE

I0454448

Empowering Seniors: Practical Strategies for Managing Stage 3 Kidney Disease with Physical Activity

Richie Smile Walker

Disclaimer

This publication is designed to provide competent and reliable information regarding the subject covered. However, the views expressed in this publication are those of the author alone, and should not be taken as expert instruction or professional advice. The reader is responsible for his or her actions. The author hereby disclaims any responsibility or liability whatsoever that is incurred from the use or application of the contents of this publication by the purchaser of the reader. The purchaser or reader is hereby responsible for his or her actions.

Table of Contents

Introduction

As our population ages, Stage 3 Kidney Disease has become a significant concern for many older individuals. This book is designed to be a helpful resource for seniors, caregivers, and healthcare professionals. Its main goal is to shed light on the crucial link between tailored exercise programs and improved kidney health, providing seniors with the necessary knowledge and tools to enhance their overall well-being and quality of life.

Throughout the book, we take a close look at the intricate details of Stage 3 Kidney Disease, aiming to help readers understand its complexities within the context of senior health. We explore various aspects of kidney function, the progression of the disease, and the potential risks and challenges that seniors with Stage 3 Kidney Disease might face.

In understanding the power of exercise, the book delves into how physical activity can significantly impact kidney health. It provides insights into low-impact exercises tailored for seniors and offers comprehensive nutritional guidelines. The book acts as a guide to help create personalized exercise routines that consider individual fitness levels and health limitations. Additionally, it discusses adaptive exercises and motivational strategies to ensure seniors can engage in physical activity safely and consistently.

Apart from exercise, the book also addresses broader lifestyle changes that can contribute to managing Stage 3 Kidney Disease effectively. It discusses stress management, the importance of regular medical check-ups, and the role of healthcare professionals in supporting exercise regimens. By covering these areas, readers can gain a comprehensive understanding of the holistic care needed for seniors with this condition.

In navigating the complexities of Stage 3 Kidney Disease and senior health, our aim is not only to provide knowledge but also to instill a sense of empowerment. By combining scientific insights with practical advice, we hope to encourage a proactive and sustainable approach to managing this condition, ultimately enabling seniors to lead vibrant and fulfilling lives.

Chapter 1:
Understanding Stage 3 Kidney Disease

Our kidneys, those small bean-shaped organs tucked away in our bodies, are unsung heroes, quietly working to keep us healthy. In this chapter, we'll take a deep dive into the world of Stage 3 Kidney Disease, aiming to shed light on its inner workings, how it progresses, and why exercise is crucial in managing it. By exploring the basics of how kidneys work, what leads to Stage 3 Kidney Disease, the risks it brings, and the importance of exercise, we'll pave the way for the following chapters, which will focus on creating exercise programs tailored for seniors dealing with this condition.

Explaining the Basics of Kidney Function

Think of your kidneys as your body's natural filtration system. They sift through your blood, removing waste and extra fluids, which then get turned into urine. But they do more than just that - they help control blood pressure, keep your electrolytes in check, and even help make red blood cells. The intricate web of nephrons inside your kidneys filters your blood and soaks up the good stuff, helping to keep your body's balance in check. Understanding this process is key to understanding how things can go awry with Stage 3 Kidney Disease.

Causes and Progression of Stage 3 Kidney Disease

Stage 3 Kidney Disease often starts with a gradual decline in kidney function, usually triggered by conditions like diabetes, high blood pressure, or certain genetic factors. During this stage, the kidney's ability to filter decreases, leading to waste buildup and fluid imbalances. If left unchecked, Stage 3 Kidney Disease can worsen, putting seniors at risk and possibly necessitating more intense treatments like dialysis or even a kidney transplant.

Risks and Complications Associated with the Disease

As Stage 3 Kidney Disease progresses, it brings with it a host of risks and complications that can seriously affect a senior's health and well-being. These can range from heart problems and anemia to bone issues, imbalances in the body's electrolytes, and an increased vulnerability to infections. The prevalence of these risks underscores the need for proactive strategies and lifestyle changes, including tailored exercise programs, to help lessen the impact of the disease and improve overall health.

Importance of Exercise in Managing Kidney Health

While the medical world has traditionally focused on treating kidney disease with medications, recent understanding highlights the critical role of exercise in comprehensive care, especially for those with Stage 3 Kidney Disease. Regular physical activity brings a range of benefits, such as improving heart health, strengthening muscles, managing weight, and boosting overall well-being. Creating exercise plans that suit the specific needs and limitations of seniors with Stage 3 Kidney Disease can help preserve kidney function and reduce associated risks.

Scope and Objectives of the Book

In this book, we aim to provide a comprehensive guide for seniors, caregivers, and healthcare professionals. We want to equip them with the necessary knowledge and practical tools to effectively integrate exercise and physical activity into the management of Stage 3 Kidney Disease. By offering insights into how kidneys work, how the disease progresses, the risks involved, and the critical role of exercise, we hope to foster a holistic understanding of the complexities of Stage 3 Kidney Disease. Our ultimate goal is to empower seniors to take proactive steps toward better kidney health and overall well-being.

Chapter 2:
Exercise and Its Impact on Kidney Health

Exercise is often hailed as a powerful tool for maintaining good health, and its benefits are especially significant for individuals dealing with Stage 3 Kidney Disease. This chapter focuses on understanding the profound effects of physical activity on kidney function, specifically tailored to the needs of seniors. By exploring the role of exercise in kidney function, highlighting the specific advantages for seniors with Stage 3 Kidney Disease, and discussing important considerations for creating exercise programs, we aim to pave the way for improved kidney health and overall well-being for this group of individuals.

Overview of the Role of Physical Activity in Kidney Function

Regular physical activity serves a multifaceted role in both preserving and enhancing kidney function. It promotes better blood circulation and oxygen delivery, facilitating efficient waste removal by the kidneys. Exercise also aids in regulating blood pressure, thereby reducing the risk of cardiovascular issues that could further complicate kidney problems. By supporting overall cardiovascular health and improving metabolic processes, exercise helps preserve kidney function and prevents further deterioration, which is particularly vital for individuals dealing with Stage 3 Kidney Disease.

Benefits of Exercise for Seniors with Stage 3 Kidney Disease

- **Improved Cardiovascular Health:** Regular exercise can significantly enhance cardiovascular health for seniors with Stage 3 Kidney Disease by strengthening the heart muscle and improving blood circulation, thus reducing the risk of associated heart complications.
- **Enhanced Muscle Strength and Flexibility:** Exercise contributes to better muscle strength and flexibility, helping seniors preserve muscle mass and improve mobility, which is crucial for managing the challenges of Stage 3 Kidney Disease.
- **Weight Management:** Exercise, when combined with a balanced diet, can effectively assist seniors in managing their weight, thereby reducing the strain on the kidneys and supporting overall health.
- **Improved Mental Well-being:** Engaging in physical activity triggers the release of endorphins, promoting a

better mood and reduced stress, which is essential for seniors coping with the emotional challenges of kidney disease.

- **Enhanced Energy Levels:** Regular exercise can combat feelings of fatigue and boost energy levels, allowing seniors to be more active in their daily lives and enhancing their overall quality of life.

- **Better Sleep Quality:** Exercise has been linked to improved sleep quality, which is essential for seniors managing Stage 3 Kidney Disease, as it contributes to better overall health and mood regulation.

- **Enhanced Bone Health:** By incorporating weight-bearing exercises and strength training, seniors can improve their bone density and reduce the risk of fractures, promoting better overall bone health.

- **Better Control of Blood Pressure:** Exercise contributes to better blood pressure control, reducing the risk of cardiovascular events and preserving kidney function in individuals with Stage 3 Kidney Disease.

- **Improved Immune Function:** Regular exercise can strengthen the immune system, reducing the susceptibility to infections and promoting better overall health for seniors dealing with compromised immune function.

- **Enhanced Overall Quality of Life:** By promoting physical well-being, mental health, and social interaction, exercise can significantly contribute to a more fulfilling and active lifestyle for seniors with Stage 3 Kidney Disease.

Considerations for Designing Exercise Programs

When creating exercise programs for seniors with Stage 3 Kidney Disease, it is crucial to have a thorough understanding of their specific health status, limitations, and individual needs. Designing exercise regimens that consider their fitness levels, mobility constraints, and any pre-existing medical conditions is essential to ensure the safety and effectiveness of the program. A well-rounded exercise plan may include low-impact aerobic exercises, flexibility routines, and strength training, all tailored to support overall well-being without placing undue stress on the kidneys. Incorporating adaptive exercises and regularly assessing progress can further ensure that seniors engage in physical activity safely and progressively, maximizing the benefits and minimizing potential risks. By adopting a personalized and holistic approach, exercise programs can become an integral part of the comprehensive management of Stage 3 Kidney Disease, leading to improved overall health outcomes and a better quality of life for seniors.

Chapter 3:
Tailoring Exercise Programs for Seniors with Stage 3 Kidney Disease

Crafting exercise programs for seniors dealing with Stage 3 Kidney Disease requires a thorough understanding of their specific health conditions, limitations, and individual needs. This chapter focuses on the essential elements of creating personalized exercise plans, including evaluating individual fitness levels and constraints, customizing exercise routines according to their health status, and integrating adaptive exercises tailored to their unique demands. By emphasizing these crucial factors, this chapter aims to assist caregivers, healthcare professionals, and seniors themselves in developing safe and effective exercise programs that contribute to improved kidney health and overall well-being.

Assessing Individual Fitness Levels and Limitations

Before initiating any exercise program, it is crucial to conduct a comprehensive assessment of the senior's fitness levels and any existing limitations they may have. This evaluation should encompass a thorough understanding of their cardiovascular endurance, muscle strength, flexibility, and overall physical capabilities. Additionally, it's essential to consider any other health conditions, such as hypertension or cardiovascular issues, which might affect the type and intensity of exercise suitable for them. By gaining a comprehensive understanding of the senior's physical abilities and limitations, caregivers and healthcare professionals can design exercise programs that are not only effective but also safe, ensuring overall health improvement without worsening any existing health concerns.

Customizing Exercise Routines Based on Health Status

Once the fitness levels and limitations of seniors with Stage 3 Kidney Disease are thoroughly assessed, the next step is to customize exercise routines according to their specific health status. This customization involves tailoring exercise plans that accommodate their unique requirements and medical considerations. For instance, incorporating low-impact aerobic exercises like walking or swimming can be beneficial for enhancing cardiovascular health without putting excessive pressure on the kidneys. Including strength training exercises can help improve muscle strength and bone density, ultimately leading to better physical function and overall well-being. Additionally, integrating flexibility exercises, such as stretching and yoga, can enhance joint mobility and reduce the risk of musculoskeletal complications. By adapting exercise routines to align with the specific health status of seniors with Stage 3 Kidney Disease, caregivers and healthcare professionals ensure that the exercise program promotes the best possible health outcomes and aids in managing the condition effectively.

Incorporating Adaptive Exercises for Seniors

Acknowledging the diverse and evolving needs of seniors with Stage 3 Kidney Disease, it is crucial to include adaptive exercises in their exercise programs. Adaptive exercises are specifically designed to accommodate any physical limitations, mobility issues, or chronic pain that seniors may experience. These exercises are gentle yet effective, allowing seniors to engage in physical activity comfortably and without discomfort. For instance, integrating chair exercises can facilitate strength training for seniors with limited mobility or balance issues. Similarly, water-based exercises can provide a low-impact and supportive environment for seniors dealing with joint pain or musculoskeletal conditions. By integrating adaptive exercises into the exercise program, caregivers and healthcare professionals ensure that seniors with Stage 3 Kidney Disease can safely participate in physical activities, promoting overall well-being and fostering a sense of empowerment and independence.

Chapter 4:
Low-Impact Exercises for Kidney Health

In managing Stage 3 Kidney Disease, incorporating gentle exercises tailored to the needs of seniors can greatly contribute to promoting kidney health and overall well-being. This chapter is dedicated to explaining the advantages and methods of including low-impact exercises in the daily routines of seniors dealing with Stage 3 Kidney Disease. It offers a detailed guide to low-impact aerobic exercises, advice on incorporating stretching and flexibility routines, and emphasizes the significance of strength-building exercises to enhance muscle function. By highlighting these essential elements, this chapter aims to provide caregivers, healthcare professionals, and seniors themselves with the necessary information to support improved kidney health and encourage a more active and fulfilling lifestyle.

Guide to Low-Impact Aerobic Exercises

Low-impact aerobic exercises form a fundamental part of an exercise plan tailored for seniors managing Stage 3 Kidney Disease. These exercises are designed to improve cardiovascular health without placing excessive stress on the body. Some recommended low-impact aerobic exercises include:

- **Walking:** A simple and effective exercise, walking promotes cardiovascular health and overall well-being. It can be easily incorporated into daily routines and adjusted to match varying fitness levels.

- **Cycling:** Cycling, either on a stationary bike or outdoors, is another low-impact aerobic exercise that enhances cardiovascular endurance and strengthens lower body muscles. It allows for customizable workout intensity and can be adapted to the specific capabilities and needs of seniors.

- **Swimming:** Swimming offers a full-body workout without exerting pressure on the joints, making it an ideal low-impact exercise for seniors with Stage 3 Kidney Disease. It contributes to cardiovascular health, muscle strength, and overall flexibility improvement.

- **Water Aerobics:** Water aerobics combines the benefits of aerobic exercise with the supportive properties of water. This exercise provides a low-impact, high-resistance workout, promoting improved cardiovascular health and enhanced muscle tone.

Incorporating Stretching and Flexibility Routines

In addition to low-impact aerobic exercises, integrating stretching and flexibility routines is crucial for seniors dealing with Stage 3 Kidney Disease. These exercises assist in enhancing joint mobility, reducing the risk of injury, and improving overall physical function. Some recommended stretching and flexibility routines include:

- **Yoga:** Yoga focuses on gentle stretching, strengthening, and balance exercises that promote flexibility and overall well-being. It encourages mindful movement and relaxation, leading to reduced stress and enhanced mental clarity.

- **Pilates:** Pilates emphasizes controlled movements targeting specific muscle groups, promoting flexibility, core strength, and overall stability. It can be tailored to suit different fitness levels and can be particularly beneficial for seniors aiming to improve posture and muscle tone.

- **Tai Chi:** Tai Chi combines slow, deliberate movements with deep breathing techniques, promoting relaxation, balance, and flexibility. It enhances muscle strength, improves posture, and supports overall physical and mental well-being.

Strengthening Exercises for Improved Muscle Function

Incorporating strength-building exercises into the exercise regimen is essential for seniors with Stage 3 Kidney Disease. These exercises help improve muscle function, enhance mobility, and reduce the risk of musculoskeletal complications. Some recommended strengthening exercises include:

- **Resistance Training:** Resistance training, involving resistance bands or light weights, aids in improving muscle strength, endurance, and overall physical function. It can be tailored to focus on specific muscle groups and adjusted to meet individual fitness levels and limitations.
- **Bodyweight Exercises:** Bodyweight exercises, such as squats, lunges, and modified push-ups, effectively build muscle strength and promote functional

movement. They can be adapted to cater to varying fitness levels and provide a convenient and accessible means of enhancing overall muscle function.

- **Modified Weight Lifting:** Incorporating modified weight lifting exercises with lighter weights and controlled movements can help build muscle strength and improve bone density without exerting excessive strain on the body. These exercises can be customized to meet the specific needs and capabilities of seniors with Stage 3 Kidney Disease.

By guiding low-impact aerobic exercises, insights into incorporating stretching and flexibility routines, and the importance of strengthening exercises for improved muscle function, this chapter aims to offer a comprehensive approach to integrating exercise into the lives of seniors with Stage 3 Kidney Disease. By incorporating these gentle exercises, seniors can experience improved cardiovascular health, enhanced flexibility, and better muscle function, ultimately contributing to their overall well-being and quality of life.

Chapter 5:
Nutrition and Hydration for Seniors with Stage 3 Kidney Disease

Maintaining the right nutrition and hydration is crucial for seniors dealing with Stage 3 Kidney Disease. This chapter sheds light on the significant role of proper nutrition in supporting kidney health, provides essential dietary guidelines and restrictions for individuals with kidney disease, and emphasizes effective hydration strategies to maintain optimal kidney function. By addressing these critical aspects, this chapter aims to provide comprehensive guidance for caregivers, healthcare professionals, and seniors, aiming for a well-rounded approach to managing nutrition and hydration in the context of Stage 3 Kidney Disease.

The Role of Nutrition in Managing Kidney Health

Understanding how nutrition profoundly impacts overall health is key to recognizing its crucial role in managing kidney health for seniors with Stage 3 Kidney Disease. A balanced diet supports optimal kidney function by regulating fluid balance, blood pressure, and electrolyte levels. It ensures the provision of vital nutrients, such as proteins, vitamins, and minerals, necessary for maintaining muscle strength, bone health, and overall well-being. Adhering to appropriate dietary guidelines and restrictions enables seniors to effectively manage the progression of kidney disease, minimize associated complications, and promote better health outcomes.

Dietary Guidelines and Restrictions for Kidney Patients

Seniors managing Stage 3 Kidney Disease need to follow specific dietary guidelines and restrictions to prevent further deterioration of kidney function and maintain overall health. Some essential dietary considerations include:

- Sodium Restriction: Seniors should limit their intake of sodium to manage fluid retention and control blood pressure. Opting for fresh, unprocessed food seasoned with herbs and spices over processed and packaged options is recommended.
- Protein Moderation: Monitoring protein consumption is crucial to avoid straining the kidneys. Seniors should focus on high-quality, low-phosphorus protein sources like poultry, fish, and egg whites while limiting intake of red meats and processed proteins.

- Phosphorus and Potassium Management: Balancing phosphorus and potassium levels is vital. Incorporating low-phosphorus foods such as grains and fruits and limiting high-potassium foods like bananas and potatoes helps prevent mineral imbalances and ease the strain on the kidneys.

- Fluid Control: Regulating fluid intake is essential for maintaining fluid balance and preventing complications associated with fluid retention. Seniors should monitor their fluid consumption, including water, beverages, and high-water-content foods, following prescribed fluid restrictions.

- Caloric Balance: Maintaining a healthy caloric balance is crucial. Seniors must balance energy intake with energy expenditure to ensure adequate nutrition while preventing excessive weight gain or loss, which can strain the kidneys.

Strategies for Effective Hydration to Support Kidney Function

In addition to following dietary guidelines and restrictions, implementing effective hydration strategies is vital for supporting kidney function and overall well-being for seniors managing Stage 3 Kidney Disease. Some crucial hydration considerations include:

- Monitoring Water Intake: Seniors should monitor their water intake to maintain optimal hydration levels without overburdening the kidneys. Tracking fluid intake and adhering to prescribed fluid restrictions can help manage fluid retention and prevent complications associated with inadequate or excessive hydration.

- Establishing Hydration Schedules: Setting up a structured hydration schedule can assist seniors in maintaining consistent fluid intake throughout the day. Having regular intervals for consuming fluids and sticking to prescribed fluid limits can support kidney function and prevent fluctuations in fluid levels, ultimately leading to better overall health outcomes.

- Choosing Suitable Fluids: Opting for hydrating options like water, herbal teas, and diluted fruit juices, and limiting the consumption of sugary beverages and caffeinated drinks is essential. These choices help seniors maintain optimal hydration levels and support kidney function.

- Recognizing Dehydration Symptoms: Being aware of dehydration symptoms and taking timely action is crucial. Seniors should monitor signs such as dry mouth, dark urine, and dizziness to identify dehydration early and take necessary steps to rehydrate, preventing potential complications and supporting overall kidney health.

Chapter 6:
Overcoming Challenges and Obstacles in Exercise

In the journey of integrating exercise into the lives of seniors managing Stage 3 Kidney Disease, various hurdles may arise. This chapter aims to address these challenges and provide effective strategies to overcome them. Focusing on dealing with fatigue and low energy levels, managing pain and discomfort during physical activity, and implementing motivational strategies for consistent exercise, this chapter serves as a guide for caregivers, healthcare professionals, and seniors themselves, fostering a supportive environment for sustained physical activity.

Dealing with Fatigue and Low Energy Levels

Seniors managing Stage 3 Kidney Disease often experience fatigue and low energy levels, making regular exercise challenging. To overcome these obstacles, it is essential to implement the following strategies:

- **Setting Realistic Goals:** Seniors should gradually increase physical activity levels, starting with achievable targets that align with their energy levels.

- **Planning Rest Periods:** Incorporating regular breaks into the exercise routine is crucial to prevent excessive fatigue and burnout.
- **Opting for Low-Intensity Workouts:** Engaging in gentle activities such as stretching and leisurely walks can help combat fatigue while promoting physical activity.

Managing Pain and Discomfort during Physical Activity

Seniors may encounter pain and discomfort during exercise, complicating consistent physical activity. Effective strategies include:

- **Consulting Healthcare Professionals:** Seeking guidance from healthcare providers can provide valuable insights into managing pain during exercise.
- **Choosing Low-Impact Exercises:** Opting for activities that are gentle on the joints, such as swimming and cycling, can help minimize discomfort.
- **Incorporating Proper Warm-ups and Cool-downs:** Implementing thorough warm-up and cool-down routines can prevent muscle strain and reduce exercise-related pain.

Motivational Strategies for Consistent Exercise

Sustaining an exercise regimen can be challenging for seniors managing Stage 3 Kidney Disease. Key motivational approaches include:

- **Establishing Support Networks:** Involving friends, family, or support groups can foster motivation and encouragement.
- **Setting Milestones and Rewards:** Acknowledging personal achievements can reinforce the importance of maintaining a consistent exercise routine.
- **Exploring Varied Exercise Options:** Trying different activities such as group exercise classes or outdoor walking clubs can keep seniors engaged and motivated.

Chapter 7:
Lifestyle Changes for Improved Kidney Health

When it comes to seniors dealing with Stage 3 Kidney Disease, making significant lifestyle changes is key. This chapter delves into various lifestyle adjustments, shedding light on stress management's impact on kidney function, the importance of healthy habits beyond exercise, strategies for maintaining overall well-being, the significance of regular medical check-ups, effective communication with healthcare professionals, and the role of physical therapists in supporting exercise routines. By addressing these components, this chapter aims to provide a holistic approach to managing lifestyle factors and fostering a supportive environment for seniors to boost their kidney health and overall quality of life.

Stress Management and Its Impact on Kidney Function

Understanding the link between stress and kidney function is vital for seniors managing Stage 3 Kidney Disease. Chronic stress can significantly affect overall health and worsen kidney disease progression. To handle stress and support kidney health effectively, the following strategies can be implemented:

- Mindfulness Practices: Engaging in mindfulness activities such as meditation, deep breathing exercises, and yoga can reduce stress levels and promote calm and well-being.
- Stress Reduction Techniques: Using stress reduction techniques like progressive muscle relaxation and guided imagery can help alleviate anxiety and build emotional resilience.
- Lifestyle Modifications: Making lifestyle changes, such as maintaining a balanced diet, getting enough sleep, and participating in enjoyable activities, can aid stress reduction and overall well-being.

Incorporating Healthy Habits Beyond Exercise

Besides regular exercise, adopting healthy habits is crucial for seniors managing Stage 3 Kidney Disease. Embracing a holistic approach to wellness can significantly impact kidney health and overall quality of life. Some important healthy habits to consider include:

- Balanced Nutrition: Following a well-balanced diet that aligns with dietary guidelines and kidney health restrictions is crucial for managing kidney disease progression and overall health support.
- Adequate Sleep: Prioritizing sufficient sleep and establishing a regular sleep schedule can contribute to improved energy levels, mood enhancement, and better overall health.
- Stress Reduction: Using stress reduction techniques and engaging in activities that promote relaxation can foster emotional well-being and support kidney health.
- Social Engagement: Maintaining social connections and taking part in social activities can enhance the sense of belonging, reduce isolation feelings, and boost overall well-being.

Strategies for Maintaining Overall Well-being

Promoting overall well-being is essential for seniors managing Stage 3 Kidney Disease. By implementing effective strategies for maintaining overall health, seniors can enjoy improved quality of life and better kidney health. Some key strategies to consider include:

- Emotional Support: Seeking emotional support from friends, family, or support groups can provide valuable encouragement and foster a sense of belonging and emotional well-being.

- Holistic Wellness Programs: Participating in holistic wellness programs that integrate components such as nutrition education, stress management, and exercise can promote overall well-being and support kidney health.

- Leisure Activities: Engaging in leisure activities and hobbies that bring joy and fulfillment can contribute to improved mental and emotional well-being, promoting a more satisfying and fulfilling lifestyle.

Importance of Regular Medical Check-ups for Kidney Health

Giving priority to regular medical check-ups is crucial for seniors managing Stage 3 Kidney Disease. Monitoring kidney function and overall health through routine medical evaluations can help identify any changes or complications early and allow timely interventions. By emphasizing the importance of regular medical check-ups, seniors can effectively manage their condition and promote better kidney health. Some essential aspects to consider include:

- Monitoring Kidney Function: Regularly monitoring kidney function through blood tests and urine analysis can help track any changes in kidney health and identify potential complications early.

- Managing Comorbidities: Addressing comorbidities such as diabetes and hypertension through regular check-ups can contribute to better overall health outcomes and support kidney health.

- Medication Management: Reviewing and adjusting medication regimens through regular medical check-ups can ensure optimal management of kidney disease and associated complications, reducing the risk of adverse health outcomes.

Communicating with Physicians and Specialists

Establishing open and effective communication with physicians and specialists is vital for seniors managing Stage 3 Kidney Disease. Building a collaborative relationship with healthcare professionals can facilitate comprehensive care and support better kidney health. By emphasizing the importance of communication, seniors can actively participate in their healthcare journey and make informed decisions regarding their well-being. Some key communication strategies to consider include:

- Sharing Concerns and Symptoms: Openly communicating any concerns, symptoms, or changes in health status with healthcare professionals can facilitate timely interventions and promote better overall health outcomes.

- Asking Questions: Engaging in meaningful conversations with physicians and specialists and asking relevant questions can provide seniors with a better understanding of their condition and empower them to make informed decisions regarding their health.

- Seeking Clarification: Seeking clarification on any medical information or treatment plans can help seniors gain a comprehensive understanding of their healthcare management and ensure that they are actively involved in their treatment journey.

Role of Physical Therapists in Supporting Exercise Routines

The role of physical therapists is crucial in supporting exercise routines and promoting overall well-being for seniors managing Stage 3 Kidney Disease. By collaborating with physical therapists, seniors can receive tailored guidance and support to enhance their exercise regimens and improve their physical function. Some essential roles that physical therapists can play in supporting exercise routines include:

- Assessing Physical Function: Conducting comprehensive assessments of physical function can help physical therapists identify any limitations or challenges that seniors may face and develop appropriate exercise plans tailored to their unique needs.

- Providing Exercise Guidance: Offering personalized exercise guidance and recommendations can assist seniors in performing exercises safely and effectively, promoting improved physical function and overall well-being.

- Monitoring Progress: Regularly monitoring and evaluating seniors' progress through exercise programs can help physical therapists track any improvements and make necessary adjustments to optimize the exercise regimen and promote better health outcomes.

Chapter 8:

30 Days Exercise Plan for Seniors with Kidney Disease

Below is a 30-day exercise plan designed for seniors managing kidney disease. This plan is tailored to accommodate various fitness levels and includes low-impact exercises, flexibility routines, and strength-building activities:

Day 1-5:

- 10 minutes of brisk walking or marching in place
- 5 minutes of gentle stretching exercises focusing on major muscle groups
- 5 minutes of deep breathing or relaxation techniques

Day 6-10:

- 15 minutes of low-impact aerobic exercises such as stationary cycling or water aerobics
- 5 minutes of yoga or tai chi to improve flexibility and balance
- 5 minutes of cool-down stretches and relaxation

Day 11-15:

- 10 minutes of swimming or water exercises for a full-body workout with reduced joint impact
- 10 minutes of resistance band exercises targeting muscle groups under the guidance of a physical therapist if needed
- 5 minutes of gentle massage or self-myofascial release using a foam roller for muscle recovery

Day 16-20:

- 15 minutes of a leisurely walk combined with arm movements for upper-body engagement
- 10 minutes of seated exercises concentrating on core strength and stability
- 5 minutes of cool-down stretches and mindfulness exercises

Day 21-25:

- 15 minutes of stationary biking or modified cycling for lower body strengthening
- 10 minutes of modified weight lifting using light dumbbells or household items for muscle toning

- 5 minutes of mindfulness exercises like meditation or deep breathing for stress reduction

Day 26-30:

- 20 minutes of combined low-impact exercises, including walking and gentle swimming
- 10 minutes of guided stretching exercises focusing on muscle flexibility
- 5 minutes of relaxation techniques and breathing exercises for mental and emotional well-being

It is essential to monitor the body's response to each exercise and adjust the plan based on individual energy levels and any physical constraints. Adequate hydration and a well-balanced diet are also critical components of this exercise plan for seniors with kidney disease.

List of Exercises for Seniors with Kidney Disease

Below is a compilation of exercises recommended for seniors managing kidney disease.

- **Brisk Walking:** A straightforward and efficient low-impact exercise suitable for indoor or outdoor settings.

- **Stationary Cycling:** An aerobic exercise that enhances cardiovascular health without causing undue stress on the joints.

- **Swimming or Water Aerobics:** Provides a thorough full-body workout with minimal impact on the joints, contributing to improved cardiovascular health and muscle strength.

- **Gentle Stretching:** A practice that aids in enhancing flexibility and reducing the likelihood of muscle stiffness and joint discomfort.

- **Yoga or Tai Chi:** Activities that promote improved flexibility, balance, and muscle strength, along with fostering relaxation and stress reduction.

- **Seated Exercises:** Designed to focus on core strength and stability, making them ideal for seniors with limited mobility.

- **Resistance Band Exercises:** A method to enhance muscle strength and endurance, with the flexibility to target specific muscle groups under the guidance of a physical therapist if necessary.

- **Modified Weight Lifting:** Utilizing light dumbbells or common household items for muscle toning and strengthening, emphasizing correct posture and controlled movements.

- **Deep Breathing Exercises:** Practices that encourage relaxation, stress reduction, and better respiratory function.
- **Meditation or Mindfulness Practices:** Techniques that support emotional well-being, reduce stress, and promote overall mental clarity and focus.

Chapter 9:

Food to Eat and Food to Avoid

List of Foods to Eat for Seniors with Kidney Disease

When seniors are managing kidney disease, being mindful of their diet becomes crucial. Here's a detailed list of foods categorized to help them plan their meals effectively:

High-Quality Protein Sources:

- Skinless poultry
- Fish, such as salmon and tuna
- Eggs
- Low-phosphorus dairy products like milk, yogurt, and cheese

Fruits and Vegetables:

- Apples
- Berries, like strawberries and blueberries
- Cabbage
- Bell peppers
- Cauliflower

- Green beans
- Eggplant

Whole Grains and Starches:

- Brown rice
- Quinoa
- Whole wheat bread
- Oatmeal

Healthy Fats:

- Olive oil
- Avocado
- Nuts, such as almonds and pistachios

Low-Potassium Foods:

- Cucumber
- Cranberries
- Grapes
- Pineapple
- Watermelon

Iron-Rich Foods:

- Red bell peppers

- Spinach
- Kale
- Broccoli

Foods Low in Sodium:

- Fresh herbs and spices
- Garlic
- Onions
- Homemade broths

Limited Phosphorus Foods:

- Unsalted popcorn
- Corn or rice cereals
- Light-colored sodas
- Light-colored fruits like peaches and pears

Foods with Low Fluid Content:

- Ice pops
- Hard candies
- Sherbet
- Jelly

Beverages:

- Herbal teas
- Fresh fruit juices (in moderation)
- Limited quantities of water to match individual fluid intake goals

List of Foods to Avoid for Seniors with Kidney Disease

When dealing with kidney disease, seniors must know which foods to avoid. Below is a categorized list to help them make informed choices when planning their meals:

Foods High in Potassium:

- Bananas
- Oranges and orange juice
- Potatoes
- Tomatoes and tomato-based products
- Avocados

Foods High in Phosphorus:

- Dairy products like cheese and milk
- Nuts and nut-based products
- Whole grains and bran

- Cola and dark sodas

Sodium-Rich Foods:

- Processed and packaged foods
- Canned soups and broths
- Deli meats and cured meats
- Pickled foods

High-Protein Foods:

- Red meat
- Processed meats like bacon and sausages
- Organ meats
- Fried or breaded meats

Foods Rich in Fluid:

- Soups and broths
- Watery fruits like watermelon and cantaloupe
- High-water-content vegetables like cucumbers and lettuce
- Gelatin desserts

Sugary Foods:

- Candies and sweets

- Sugary beverages like sodas and sweetened juices

- Pastries and baked goods with high sugar content

- Sweetened cereals and snacks

Foods with Phosphorus Additives:

- Processed foods with phosphorus-containing additives

- Colas and dark sodas

- Packaged snacks and convenience foods

- Instant or flavored rice and pasta mixes

Excessive Caffeine and Alcohol:

- Coffee and caffeinated beverages

- Alcoholic beverages

- Energy drinks and highly caffeinated teas

- Chocolate and cocoa products

Conclusion

Embracing a Healthier Lifestyle for Better Kidney Health

As we come to the end of our exploration of exercise and physical activity for seniors managing Stage 3 Kidney Disease, it's important to look back at what we've learned. This final chapter is a summary of the valuable insights and guidance provided throughout the book. It emphasizes the significance of adopting a healthy and active lifestyle to improve kidney health and overall well-being. By highlighting the key points, offering encouragement for seniors to make positive lifestyle changes, and expressing final thoughts and best wishes for enhanced kidney health, we hope to motivate and empower seniors to embark on a rewarding wellness journey.

Recapping Key Lessons from the Book

In this book, we've covered various aspects of exercise and physical activity designed for seniors dealing with Stage 3 Kidney Disease. We emphasized the importance of specific exercises, such as low-impact aerobics, stretching, and strength training, in promoting better kidney health. We also stressed the significance of maintaining a balanced diet, staying well-hydrated, and adopting lifestyle changes to effectively manage kidney health. We discussed strategies for overcoming challenges, building resilience, and sticking to consistent exercise routines. Additionally, we explored the vital roles of healthcare professionals, the importance of regular check-ups, and the support offered by physical therapists in facilitating exercise regimens. These key takeaways contribute to a holistic approach to managing kidney disease and promote a more active and fulfilling lifestyle for seniors.

Encouraging Seniors to Adopt a Healthy and Active Lifestyle

As we conclude, it is crucial to encourage seniors to fully embrace a healthy and active lifestyle. By prioritizing regular exercise, following appropriate dietary guidelines, and incorporating positive lifestyle changes, seniors can make significant strides in improving their kidney health and overall quality of life. Seniors need to approach their wellness journey with a positive mindset, determination, and resilience. Engaging in activities that bring joy, nurturing relationships, and seeking guidance from healthcare professionals can provide the necessary motivation for seniors to embark on a transformative path toward better health and well-being.

Final Thoughts and Best Wishes for Improved Kidney Health

In closing, we extend our heartfelt best wishes to all seniors managing Stage 3 Kidney Disease. Your commitment to prioritizing your health and well-being is commendable, and your dedication to embracing positive lifestyle changes is truly inspiring. Remember that every small step you take toward a healthier lifestyle contributes to your overall well-being and vitality. Approach this journey with optimism and determination, knowing that consistent efforts, no matter how small, can lead to significant improvements in your kidney health and overall quality of life. May your days be filled with energy, joy, and a renewed sense of purpose as you continue to nurture your body, mind, and spirit. Here's to better kidney health, increased resilience, and a life filled with health, happiness, and fulfillment.